MW01046977

Balancing Screen Time: A Guide for Parents.

By Amanda Coppin

Contents

Dedication

I would like to thank the Almighty God for supporting me through the high and lows of my life. To my husband Viktor and daughters Apolla and Montega, who have stuck with me on our journey and been inspirations and motivation to write this book. To my brother & sister-in-law and nephew who have always been there for support. My late mother and father who have shown me how to love and be a parent and finally to my foster children who have tested my skills and patients to continue to shape my growth and development as a parent/carer.

To all of them I give great thanks.

This book is also dedicated to all parents and families out there who arc struggling with their children, husbands or wives to the additive powers of technology.

Chapter 1

Welcome to Balancing Screen Time: A Guide for Parents.

Firstly, well done for taking this first step on your journey towards a more balanced and fulfilling family life. Because I promise that's what managing screen time will give you. While screens are a vital aspect of modern parenting, it can be challenging. But by understanding the potential impacts of excessive screen use and implementing practical strategies to reduce it, you're already moving closer towards a healthier, more balanced lifestyle for you and your children.

In today's digital age, screens are an integral part of our daily lives, offering both benefits and challenges, especially for young children. As parents, we're all striving to find a balance that ensures our children reap the educational and entertainment benefits of technology while protecting them from its potential pitfalls. Achieving this as a home educating mother and foster parent with six children in my care has been incredibly challenging. But with some pitfalls along the way, we found a formula that worked for us. The practical advice I share in this book is based on my journey,

It's designed to help you navigate the complexities of screen time of all types for your children, providing practical strategies, engaging alternatives, and valuable insights. Whether you're concerned about the impact of screens on your child's health or looking for ways to enrich their development with non-screen activities, this book offers a comprehensive approach to creating a balanced and healthy screen environment in your home.

Our family tech purge: before and after

Before fostering, we made the choice to home educate our children and take them out of what we saw as an increasingly restrictive and counterproductive full time education system. We also started clearing our home from tech by getting rid of our television when they were ten and seven. This may seem like a crazy idea for many families, but for us we noticed a dependency that we weren't comfortable with which caused many heated debates.

For example, Most mornings before school The TV would miraculously turn on and they would be watching TV whilst eating breakfast. This would end up causing them to be sucked into the programmes, which meant they were unable to get on with what they needed to do before leaving for school. Causing us to often be late or having to run down the road to get to school on time.

I have often visited friends and family who have children and my children often complain that they have no ability to play or have conversations as they just want to share things with them from their phones or just glued to their gaming screens. Within my home when we have guests and visitors, phones are often confiscated from teens and board games or card games come out instead. This often leads to hours of fun had by all.

I have witnessed many more babies and toddlers in pushchairs on the phones rather than then looking around and being spoken to by their parents carer. This also happens in many restaurants where children are not engaged in conversation but plugged into their tablets even when the food arrives. This means that we are raising these children to struggle socially as they are not being exposed to these situations and learning from them.

Finally I have seen many families breaking down due to the fact that everyone in the house is on a device and no one is interacting with the others. Mum & Dad may be catching up on work that they missed due to meetings and the children may be scrolling through one of the many social media apps like Tik Tok, Instagram or chat via Snapchat or Whatsapp. If family time was family time where parents didn't have to bring their work home and children had a space to offload their thoughts and emotions of the day, I think many families would be stronger and happier.

Life now is calmer and very different. We live in a house with a TV that is used as a computer monitor. We all collectively watch one or two films a week and after school the children go on computers for a maximum of half an hour for homework (most schools no longer encourage children to write and research from books or send home paper homework, but expect the children to complete paid educational programmes like Educake, Times Tables Rockstars and Sparx Maths on their computer.

I believe that children should use a pen and paper everyday to maintain and develop their fine motor skills and develop their handwriting. My children write a story or copy from a book and they do some maths work even through the holidays.

I now have an 18-year-old who uses a mobile phone and laptop to run and manage her own business. I have two 15-year-olds who have access to a phone, one has a nokia brick for going to and from school and one uses my spare mobile phone for supporting the family business in posting Tik Toks and sending messages to customers. They don't have their own phones which significantly reduces arguments as the phones belong to me as their parent and they are allowed to use them for set times and tasks.

I also have children of 11, 9 and 8 who have laptops for homework.

Why are we letting our children use screens so much?

We've all seen the social commentary on lazy parents ignoring their children by shoving a device in their hands, but in reality, parents use screens for their young children for a variety of reasons, ranging from educational purposes to convenience. Here are the eight most common:

1. **Educational content and learning tools**: Parents use screens to provide access to educational programs, apps, and games that can support early learning, language development, and cognitive skills. They're used to supplement traditional learning with interactive and engaging content that reinforces educational concepts taught at home or in preschool settings.

2. **Keeping children occupied**: Screens are commonly used to entertain children and keep them engaged, especially in situations where parents need to focus on other tasks or manage household responsibilities.

3. **Calming and soothing**: Screens are often used to calm and soothe children, particularly during stressful moments or when they're upset.

4. **Social interaction**: Parents use screens to facilitate video calls with family members and friends, helping children maintain social connections with loved ones who are not physically present.

5. **Behaviour management**: Screens are sometimes used as part of a reward system, granted as a reward for good behaviour or completing tasks.

6. **Routine and structure**: Screens can be integrated into daily routines, such as watching a favourite show at a specific time, providing a sense of structure and predictability for children.

7. **Exposure to technology**: Parents use screens to familiarise their children with technology, helping them develop basic tech skills that are increasingly important in the modern world.

8. All round use including taking pictures, using the calendar, calculator and internet searching.

While these reasons and uses can offer benefits, which I'll explore in the book, it's important for parents to monitor and regulate screen time to ensure it is balanced with other essential activities and interactions.

Chapter 2.

Understanding screen time and its impact

Understanding screen time and its effects is crucial for parents, educators, and policymakers to make informed decisions about the use of digital devices by children.

In today's digital age, screen time has become an integral part of our daily lives. From smartphones and tablets to computers and televisions, screens are everywhere, but while technology has brought about numerous benefits, such as enhanced communication, educational resources, and entertainment, it has also raised concerns, particularly regarding its impact on children. This chapter explores the concept of screen time, its impact on children in different age groups (0-3 years, 4-7 years, and 7+ years), and the importance of limiting screen time to promote healthy development.

0-3 years

The brain undergoes rapid cognitive, emotional, and social development during this critical period, with sensory experiences and interactions with caregivers playing a <u>VITAL ROLE</u>. Excessive screen time can interfere with these essential interactions. The American Academy of Paediatrics (AAP) recommends NO SCREEN time for children under 18 months, except for video chatting. For children aged 18-24 months, screen time should be limited to high-quality programming with parental involvement. **Personally, I would not recommend any access to a screen for a 0-3 year-old unless it involves speaking to someone over the phone. I also believe that anything to do with counting and singing should involve us, as parents and caregivers.**

Potential health issues from prolonged screen use

- **Developmental concerns**: Young children learn best through hands-on activities and real-life interactions and screens provide passive stimuli, which can detract from time spent exploring the physical world and engaging with caregivers. Excessive screen time in this age group can delay language acquisition, impair social skills, and reduce the quality of sleep.

- **Behavioural issues**: Prolonged screen use can lead to attention problems and increased irritability. Children who are exposed to fast-paced and overstimulating content may find it challenging to focus on slower-paced, real-world activities.

- **Vision problems**: Staring at screens for extended periods can cause eye strain and discomfort, known as Computer Vision Syndrome. For infants and toddlers, this can be particularly concerning as their eyes are still developing.

- **Sleep disruption**: Screen time, especially before bedtime, can interfere with sleep. The blue light emitted by screens can suppress melatonin production, making it harder for young children to fall asleep and stay asleep.

- **Attention deficits**: Prolonged exposure to fast-paced, high-stimulation content can affect attention spans and increase the risk of attention-deficit disorders. Young children are particularly vulnerable as their brains are highly malleable.

0-5 years

The impact of screen time on children aged 0-5 years is a topic of considerable interest and ongoing research. Here are some of the

8

positive and negative effects of screen use for more than an hour a day in this age group:

All screen time should be supervised, so that carers can help make sense of what the child is watching. Not all child content is suitable for children as there are many examples of popular children content that has been dubbed with foul language or unsuitable visuals may be inserted into the centre without your knowledge.

Negative effects

Cognitive development

- **Attention issues**: Excessive screen time, especially passive consumption, has been linked to attention problems and decreased ability to concentrate.

- **Delayed language development**: Overuse of screens, particularly if it replaces interactive, conversational activities, can lead to delays in language acquisition.

Physical health

- **Sleep disruption**: Screen exposure, especially before bedtime, or in the bedroom, can interfere with sleep patterns due to the stimulating content and blue light emitted by screens. Most sleep experts recommend not having TVs in bedrooms, due to the electric magnetic fields.

- **Obesity**: Prolonged screen time is associated with a sedentary lifestyle, which can contribute to childhood obesity.

Social and emotional development

- **Reduced face-to-face interaction**: Excessive screen use can decrease the amount of direct human interaction, which is crucial for social skills development.

- **Emotional regulation**: Over reliance on screens for soothing or entertainment can impede the development of self-regulation skills.

Behavioural Issues

- **Aggressive behaviour**: Exposure to violent content can lead to increased aggression and behavioural problems in young children.

- **Dependency**: Excessive screen time can lead to screen dependency, where children may have difficulty engaging in non-screen activities.

4-7 years

Children aged 4-7 years are in the early stages of formal education and their cognitive, social, and emotional skills continue to develop rapidly. While screens can be educational, it is essential to balance screen time with other activities that promote physical health, creativity, and social interaction. I would recommend no longer than 1hr a week broken into 3x20 minute chunks

Potential health issues from prolonged screen use

- **Obesity**: Sedentary behaviour associated with prolonged screen time can lead to weight gain and obesity. Lack of physical activity, combined with snacking while watching screens, can exacerbate this issue.

- **Behavioural problems**: Excessive screen time has been linked to behavioural issues such as aggression and defiance. Exposure to violent or inappropriate content can influence behaviour and desensitise children to violence.

- **Reduced physical fitness**: Developing motor skills and overall physical health requires regular physical activity, which is often compromised by excessive screen use. Physical inactivity due to screen time can result in poor physical fitness.

- **Cognitive development**: Educational programs and apps can support learning, but excessive screen time can hinder the development of critical thinking and problem-solving skills. Interactive and imaginative play is crucial for cognitive growth during this period.

- **Physical health**: Physical activities such as outdoor play and sports are essential for developing motor skills and maintaining a healthy weight. Prolonged screen use can contribute to sedentary behaviour, increasing the risk of obesity and related health issues.

- **Social skills**: Children in this age group need to engage in face-to-face interactions to develop social skills, empathy, and emotional regulation. Excessive screen time can reduce opportunities for socialisation and lead to difficulties in forming and maintaining relationships.

7+ years

As children grow older, their use of screens for educational purposes increases. However, it's crucial to monitor and limit recreational screen time to ensure a healthy balance between digital and non-digital activities. I would recommend a maximum of 2 hrs a week. Ideally broken into 2x 1 hr sessions.

Potential issues from prolonged screen use

- **Mental health issues**: Overuse of social media and online gaming can lead to mental health problems such as anxiety, depression, and social withdrawal. Cyberbullying and exposure to inappropriate content are also significant concerns in this age group.

- **Poor academic performance**: Excessive recreational screen time can interfere with homework, reading, and other educational activities. This can negatively impact academic performance and reduce overall academic achievement.

- **Sleep problems**: Like younger children, older children and adolescents can also experience sleep disturbances due to screen use, particularly if they use screens before bedtime. Blue light emitted by screens can disrupt sleep patterns, leading to insufficient rest. Poor sleep quality can affect mood, cognitive function, and overall health

- **Academic performance**: While educational technology can enhance learning, excessive recreational screen time can negatively impact academic performance. It's essential for children to prioritise homework, reading, and other educational activities over screen-based entertainment. However, homework is increasing on computers.

Additional physical health issues that can affect all age groups, including adults

Vision problems

- **Digital eye strain**: Extended screen use can cause eye strain, discomfort, and fatigue, often referred to as "digital eye strain" or "computer vision syndrome."

- **Myopia (nearsightedness)**: Increased screen time, particularly with devices held close to the eyes, has been linked to a higher risk of developing myopia.

Obesity

- **Unhealthy eating habits**: Screen time, particularly during meals, can lead to mindless eating and an increased intake of unhealthy snacks and sugary drinks.

Poor posture and musculoskeletal issues

- **Postural problems**: Spending long periods in front of screens can lead to poor posture, which may cause neck, back, and shoulder pain.

- **Repetitive strain injuries**: Frequent use of handheld devices and keyboards can cause repetitive strain injuries in the hands, wrists, and arms.

Positive effects for all age groups with limited exposure to screens

Educational content

- **Learning opportunities**: High-quality educational programs and apps can support language development, cognitive skills, and early literacy if used interactively and under adult supervision.

- **Exposure to diverse concepts**: Screens can introduce children to a wide range of ideas and cultures, expanding their understanding of the world.

Interactive learning

- **Engagement**: Interactive media can engage children in ways that encourage learning through play, such as problem-solving games and interactive storybooks.

- **Motor skills**: Certain apps and games can help develop fine motor skills through activities that require precise movements. However this does not beat Physical tasks like holding and using pencils, or playing with small objects as well as counting small objects like grapes or rice.

Social interaction

- **Video calls**: Screen time through video calls can help young children maintain relationships with distant family members, contributing to their social development.

- **Development of time management:** When children have their allocated time on the screen, parents should put a phone timer or cooker timer on to let everyone know when time is up. If a child is indecisive on what they want to watch/play then they use up all their time searching.

Parents can help children plan by asking them before they start what are you going to do or watch and even find it before the child starts. No extra time should be given at all.

Chapter 3.

Take control: A step-by-step approach to breaking the cycle of excessive screen usage

Assessing current screen usage

Given the ubiquity of screens in modern life, it's easy to lose track of how much time is spent in front of devices. Before making any changes in yours or your children's screen usage I would suggest you take a week to monitor and review what their normal behaviours are so that the changes can be based on the evidence from this week. Remember to capture all screens from Tv's, Game consoles, phones, tablets, laptops. When assessing please try to be neutral and refrain from casing judgement on what and how much you see. Getting a true reflection of usage is the most important thing.

The first thing you can do is set the phone to "monitor your usage" under the Digital Wellbeing and parental controls. To do this:

1. Go into the setting on your phone

2. Go to Digital wellbeing and parental controls

3. Go through and turn things on so that it can begin to monitor your usage of all apps

4. Remember, do not set any limits or timers at this time

At the end of each day, add the information into the chart below:

Date	Duration	Device	Activity	Reason	Notes

Observing and logging screen time

For this chart, we'll need to gather data over a period (e.g. one week) and log details such as the time of day, the duration of screen usage, the device used, the activity performed, and the reason for using the screen. We'll then analyse this data to identify patterns and reasons for screen use.

Here's an outline of how the chart could be structured:

Date	Time of day	Duration (minutes)	Device	Activity	Reason for use
2024-07-16	08:00 - 09:00	60	Smartphone	Social Media	Habit
2024-07-16	10:00 - 11:00	30	Laptop	Work	Professional need
2024-07-16	13:00 - 13:30	30	Tablet	Reading	Leisure
2024-07-16	20:00 - 21:00	60	Television	Watching TV Show	Entertainment
...	...	...	...	...	...

This chapter outlines the key questions, key steps to help with your goal setting, How to create and manage the transition to less screens in your life.

Goals can be set to be completed by a set date with a gradual reduction leading to that date, using some of the strategies I've included in this chapter. This should be done by all adults, and older children who may care for younger siblings as they are the leaders of the family and should at all times set an example.

Your goal may be: to spend more time together as a family,

to increase the safety of your children while they are online,

reduce your children's dependency on technology, (improve mental health)

to develop better relationships with your children, (teach them through conversation and life)

to control the images, films, videos that your children are being exposed to. (maintain their hearts and minds for a long as possible)

Questions to ask yourself and family before you set your goal:

- Will you be getting rid of the TV?

- Will you only watch TV on weekends?

- Will you take out all the tv and playstation from the childrens rooms?

- Will you be able to stop using your phone at a set time everyday ie 7pm phone get put away to charge?

- What activities will you do instead?

- Where will phones be stored? a lockable cabinet?

- Is your mobile your main communication with the outside world? If so, place it somewhere that is still accessible.

- What do you hope to achieve by doing this? More connection with family, less separation?

- What would be the exceptions?

- How do you plan to review your progress and how often?

- Would you all move all technology down out of bedrooms?

- Do you receive and make many calls to family in the evening? If so they would need to know about the new plan so that they can support you?

- Will you need to purchase alarm clocks/ watches/camera?

In the run up to your agreed date, I'd encourage you to have discussions and make plans with all members of the family, with a shared understanding that on the agreed date everything changes. You can plant the idea of having more time to play, talk and spend time together and then an excitement can be built up to the change date. This can even include a countdown and a party on the first night of screen free time.

The aim should be clear: to get all individuals of screens and devices by a set time so that the family can play games together, have discussions or do an activity like painting, clay making or planning a holiday/ adventure.

To ensure a balanced lifestyle, parents and caregivers must set appropriate goals for screen time reduction and create a daily schedule that fits the needs of each child, depending on their age and developmental stage.

Key steps -

Set the family goal, decide on a date. Choose a method, have discussions and do it.

Methods

1. Cold turkey- this is the more abrupt method which could cause the most backlash from young members of the family, but it's like ripping a plaster off a cut. It will sting but the result for healing will happen quicker.

2. The second approach is the gradual reduction method which can happen over a longer period of time 6-12 weeks. This requires more work and attention on the parents' part as they have to be consistent, diligent and positive about the changes that are happening.

3. One area at a time: If you have decided that many areas need to be changed but the first 2 options may be too swift or may cause it to be unsettling for members of your family. I would suggest you make a plan of deleting tech every month or 2 months over the year.

Making it happen: Tactics for weaning off screens

Well done! You've set your goal and have a plan, but how will it work in practice?

We all know that breaking long-standing habits is incredibly hard and weaning a child/adult off excessive screen time requires a gradual and supportive approach. There is no easy solution, but by sticking to your plan and sticking together, you *can* strike a balance between the benefits of digital technology and the importance of real-world interactions and activities.

Here are the steps, including time frames, verbal prompts, and tools, needed to help reduce screen time to one hour a day:

Your step-by-step plan

Assess current usage (Week 1)

- **Observation**: Track and log your child's current screen time and identify patterns. Use a stopwatch to see how long they are on their devices. Note when and why the screen is used most. You can use the screen assessment form in chapter 3.

Set clear goals and create a schedule (Week 2)

- **Establish the ultimate goal**:(e.g. 30 mins -1 hour of screen time per day.

- **Create a schedule**: Develop a daily schedule that includes specific times for screen use and other activities

- **Discussion**: Ask your children what fun non computer fun activities would they like to start doing. Make a list and separate those that cost and those that are free. These can be put in separate jars to use later when screen time reduces.

If you have a neurodiverse child or a child who struggles with change, use the plan but reduce the timing so it's more gentle.

- Jan - Reduce time on Laptops for homework- research library use books

- March - Reduce gaming time - Increase activities together

- May - get rid of TVs in bedrooms- rearrange, redecorate or deep clean

Gradual reduction (week 3)

: Reduce screen time by 15 minutes each day in the evening.

- o **Verbal prompt**: "We have some exciting new activities planned! we can do screens later"

- o **Activity substitution**: Introduce one or two new activities during the time that was previously used for screens

- o **Discussion**: Let the child know that this week is the start of us doing more fun things together.

- **(Week 4)** Further reduce screen time by another 30 minutes.

  - o **Verbal prompt**: Let's play with our building blocks. We can have some screen time later."

  - o **Reinforce alternative activities**: Emphasise engaging alternatives such as outdoor play, reading, or arts and crafts

- **Week 5-6**: Continue reducing screen time until it reaches the target of one/two hours a week

  - o **Verbal prompt**: "We're going to have so much fun playing outside and reading a book!"

  - o **Establish routines**: Make non-screen activities a consistent part of the daily routine - play cards, hangman, scrabble, colouring and whatever other activities your child likes or you can think of.

4. **Maintain consistency and monitor (ongoing)**

- **Consistency**: Stick to the established screen time schedule and continue offering a variety of alternative activities. Please do not crumble when they beg, cry or argue. This is all for their health and wellbeing.

- **Monitoring**: Regularly review and adjust the schedule as needed to ensure it fits well with the child's needs and family dynamics

- ALWAYS DO FUN ACTIVITY FIRST THEN SCREENS THEN DINNER!

Other recommendations

To mitigate the negative effects of screen use and enhance positive ones, consider the following guidelines:

- **Set clear guidelines**: Establish clear rules for screen time, including limits on daily use and restrictions on the type of content that can be accessed. Consistency is key to ensuring that children understand and adhere to these guidelines

- **Encourage other activities**: Promote regular physical activity by scheduling screen-free times for outdoor play, sports, and other physical activities. This is crucial for maintaining a healthy weight and developing motor skills. Encouraging children to engage in a variety of other activities, such as reading, playing with toys, arts and crafts, and spending time with family and friends, will also help to develop a well-rounded set of skills and interests

- **Model healthy behaviour**: Parents and caregivers should model healthy screen habits by limiting their own screen time and engaging in screen-free activities with their children. This sets a positive example and reinforces the importance of balance

- **Create screen-free zones**: Designate certain areas of the home, such as bedrooms and dining areas, as screen-free zones. This encourages face-to-face interactions and reduces the likelihood of screens interfering with sleep and meals

- **Prioritise educational content**: Choose high-quality, educational content that aligns with the child's developmental stage. Co-viewing and discussing the content can enhance learning and ensure that screen time is meaningful

Alternatives to screen time

If you're looking for alternatives to screen time there are many options that can support development, learning, and play. The following suggestions not only provide diverse opportunities for learning and development but also promote healthy habits and strong family connections:

Reading and story time

- Reading books aloud to children supports language development, imagination, and bonding. Interactive books with flaps, textures, and sounds can be particularly engaging for young children.

Outdoor play: Encouraging outdoor play helps children develop motor skills, explore their environment, and engage in physical exercise. Activities can include playing in the park, riding tricycles, or simply running around. This also supports their bodies production of vitamin D from being outdoors in the sun.

Creative arts and crafts: Providing materials for drawing, painting, colouring, and crafting can stimulate creativity and fine motor skills. Simple projects like making collages, playdough modelling, or finger painting are great options.

Music and dance: Singing songs, playing simple musical instruments, and dancing to music can be fun and educational. Music activities help with rhythm, coordination, and auditory skills.

Problem-solving toys: Engaging with puzzles, building blocks, and other manipulative toys supports cognitive development, spatial awareness, and fine motor skills.

Imaginative play: Encouraging pretend play with dolls, action figures, toy kitchens, and dress-up clothes fosters creativity, social skills, and language development.

Nature exploration: Taking children on nature walks, gardening, or exploring local parks and trails can be a great way to learn about the natural world and develop curiosity.

Sensory play: Providing sensory play activities such as sandboxes, water tables, sensory bins filled with rice or beans, and textured toys can engage children's senses and support sensory development.

Family games and activities: Playing simple board games, card games, or engaging in family-friendly activities like treasure hunts can promote family bonding and teach children social skills and turn-taking.

Social interaction: Enrolling children in structured activities such as story time at the library, toddler gym classes, music groups, or playdates with peers provides social interaction and developmental benefits.

Library day: This can help teens do research for their homework without a screen

Additional tools and support

Visual timers:

- Use visual timers to help the child understand how much screen time is left and when it will end.

Reward system:

- Implement a reward system to reinforce positive behaviour. For example, use a sticker chart to track successful days without exceeding screen time.

Parental controls:

- Utilise parental controls on devices to limit screen time automatically and block inappropriate content. There are also apps that allow parents to turn off phone remotely and see what their child is doing like - Aura · 2. Qustodio · 3. Net Nanny. Please do some research and choose the one that suits your needs.

Modelling Behaviour:

- Set a positive example by reducing your own screen time and engaging in alternative activities with your child. Therefore if you are using your screen at the same time as your child is using the screen when their time has finished you should finish too.

Support Network:

- Involve other caregivers and family members in the plan to ensure consistent messaging and support.

Verbal prompts and encouragement

- **Positive reinforcement**: "You did a great job playing outside today instead of watching TV. I'm so proud of you!"

- **Redirection**: "Let's finish this game and then we can read your favourite book."

- **Encouragement**: "I know you love your screen time, but there are so many other fun things we can do together!"

Dealing with resistance

1st allow screen time in between an activity and a meal. Make the activity lots of fun and they will not want to stop the screen time. Always let them have the choice to stop the fun activity to go on the screens and explain that they will miss it or it will be to late for it.

- **Stay calm**: Remain patient and calm if your child resists the changes.

- **Acknowledge feelings**: Validate their feelings by saying, "I know it's hard to turn off the screen, but let's try something new and fun together."

- **Gradual changes**: If the child struggles, slow down the reduction process slightly to give them more time to adjust.

By following these steps, providing engaging alternatives, and offering consistent support and encouragement, you can help your children transition to a healthier balance of screen time and other activities.

Family time, including mealtime

Replacing screen use, particularly at mealtimes, with engaging, family-oriented activities can enhance communication, bonding, and overall wellbeing. Here are several alternatives to screen use when you're together as a family:

Conversation starters

- **Family stories**: Share stories about family history or funny anecdotes from the past

- **Daily highlights**: Ask each family member to share the best part of their day or something they learned

Interactive games

- **Tabletop games**: Simple, quick games like "I Spy," "20 Questions," "Guess the Animal" or would you rather can make mealtimes fun and interactive

- **Word association**: Start with a word, and each person takes turns saying a word related to the previous one

Educational activities

- **Fun facts**: Share interesting facts about the food you're eating, such as its origin, nutritional benefits, or how it's grown

- **Quiz time**: Create a short quiz on various topics to engage everyone's minds

Creative activities

- **Storytelling**: Make up a story together, with each person adding a sentence or two

- **Drawing and colouring**: Provide paper and crayons or coloured pencils for children to draw or colour while waiting for their meal

Mindfulness practices

- **Gratitude circle**: Each person shares something they are grateful for in their lives or about someone else in the family.

- **Mindful eating**: Encourage everyone to focus on the taste, texture, and smell of their food, promoting a mindful eating experience, this could be done blindfolded or with nose plugs.

Learning about food

- **Recipe discussions**: Talk about the recipes used for the meal and involve children in planning future meals

- **Food exploration**: Introduce new foods and discuss their flavours, textures, and cultural significance

Family planning

- **Schedule review**: Discuss upcoming family plans, events, or activities

- **Menu planning**: Involve children in planning the menu for the week, encouraging them to make healthy choices

Music and singing

- **Background music**: Play soft, calming music to create a pleasant dining atmosphere

- **Sing-along**: Have a family sing-along with favourite songs or nursery rhymes

Physical activities

- **Post-meal walk**: Plan a short family walk after meals to promote physical activity and digestion

- **Table exercises**: Simple stretching exercises that can be done while seated to keep young children engaged

Role-playing

- **Restaurant role-play**: Let the children decide on the meal for the next day. It could be spaghetti bolognaise, curry, fish and chips or whatever you can prepare. For two evenings they could plan the menu and bring it to life with colouring pens and paper. They can find uniforms for themselves as waiters. This will give them a chance to serve you and if they are teens then get all the ingredients and allow them to cook the meal themselves. Younger children can be servers

- **Themed meals**: Create themed meals (e.g., Italian night, picnic indoors) and dress up or decorate the table accordingly

- **Themed nights**: such as cinema night: When my children were younger they used to create tickets and move the chairs to create a movie-like atmosphere, with popcorn to finish it off

- **Disco:** The children would take over the living room and create a sign for the disco, then get the music speaker out that has a light at the top. They'd then create a 'bar' and they have one person as the door person security and the other person is a bartender

- **Theatre nights:** Children would use a well-known book that they have read and make a performance with costumes and props. This is a great activity especially when cousins or friends come around and this can take a few hours of their time.

- **Fashion shows:** The children could perform a fashion show with a range of clothes and costumes that they make themselves

- **Role playing games:** These are a great way to get the whole family involved and for them to take on different characters and personalities. For example the quieter child could be the loud complaining rich customer and the loud child has to be the quite polite manager who tried to resolve the issues. This is a great way to help them develop different social skills that they might not have yet.

Implementation tips

- **Consistency**: Make these activities a regular part of mealtimes to build a new routine. Have meals together as a family at the table.

- **Involvement**: Encourage all family members to participate and suggest new activities

- **Patience**: Be patient as children and adult adjust to the new routine without screens.

- **Preparation**: Have materials (like colouring books or quiz questions) ready before the meal begins to smoothly transition into these activities

- **Tough love**: Remember why you're making these changes

By incorporating these alternatives, family time can become a screen-free opportunity for bonding, learning, and fun.

Chapter 4

Role modelling (adults benefit from reduced screen time too!)

In this section, I explore the approaches and techniques adults can use to reduce their screen time alongside their children.

While this guide focuses on children and young people, the drawbacks of overuse of screens in adults are also well documented. The importance of role modelling a life not centred around screens is vital in making the approaches set out in this book successful. Normalising a balanced, holistic life uncontrolled by a random device is one of the most powerful things you can do for your children, so if your children see you embodying this, rather than someone who is constantly absorbed by their phone, you have a far more realistic chance of succeeding.

We all know anecdotally that even short bursts of effort to use screens have a huge impact on our mental health, time management, and much more. Which means you'll reap the benefits as well as your family.

Here are some ideas.

Identifying patterns and reasons for your screen use

Pattern	Frequency	Main Reasons	Suggested action
Morning smartphone usage	Daily	Habit, news updates	Consider setting a time limit
Work-related screen time	5 times/week	Professional need	Necessary for job
Leisure reading on tablet	3 times/week	Relaxation	Positive use of screen time
Evening TV watching	Daily	Entertainment, unwind	Balance with other activities

Using this template, you can log your daily screen time activities, then analyse them to find patterns and understand the reasons behind your screen use. This helps in identifying areas where you might want to reduce screen time or change habits for better balance and well-being.

To visualise this data, a bar chart or pie chart can be created to represent the duration of screen time for each category, and a line graph can show screen usage trends over the week.

Now you can go to settings on the phone to "monitor your usage" under the Digital Wellbeing and parental controls. To do this:

5. Go into the setting on your phone

6. Go to Digital wellbeing and parental controls

7. Go through all apps and turn on the timers based on your reduction plan.

8. This can be adjusted to help you with time as you may need to be off social media and spend more time on whatsapp as you realise that you use that more. (try to change just once a week or once a month)

Reduce your screen time when children are up so they have the chance to be with you.

Chapter 5

Conclusion

In reading this book, I'm guessing you were looking for evidence of something you already knew:

- Managing screen time is a challenging but vital aspect of modern parenting

- Engaging in diverse, enriching activities not only supports your children's development but also strengthens family bonds

Many of the people I speak to about this topic express regret at the time they have lost, or a sense of shame about any negative effects that have already occurred, but please don't be too hard on yourself. Screen time is an inevitable part of modern life which means this is an incredibly difficult journey. By making the decision to understand the potential impacts of excessive screen use and implementing practical strategies to reduce it, you immediately began to foster a healthier, more balanced lifestyle for your children. That is a huge positive.

Remember, the goal is not to eliminate screens entirely but to ensure that their use is mindful and balanced and minimises negative impact on children's development. By taking small, consistent steps and involving your children in the process, you *can* create a positive and sustainable approach to screen time, ensuring that your children grow up healthy, balanced, and well-adjusted.

Thank you for taking this journey towards a more balanced and fulfilling family life.

You can do it. I believe in you!

About the author

Amanda Coppin has been a home educating mother for ten years. For five of those years she has been a "professional parent", otherwise known as a foster parent! She has six amazing children in her care. All who have grown up with less than 1 hr a week on screens and as they grow up this amount has increased due to school work or working on the businesses.

Amanda was blessed to have children and young people in her life from a young age as her mother raised other people's children as a child minder and then she became a youth and community worker. Since having her children she has always worked for her self - running successful businesses which have included dance classes and currently an Organic Natural remedies shop called "Mamaz Organics"

This book was a part of Amanda's passion for supporting Parents and all things parenting in the hope that it helps someone improve relationships.

Made in the USA
Middletown, DE
10 January 2025

68310348R00024